Frc

Copyright

From One Mended Heart to Another

Or

The Cardiac Patient's Companion

Disclaimer: The author of this book is not a medical professional. Everything written in this book comes strictly from her own experience and observations as a cardiac patient and a visitor of many others. This book is written for encouragement and inspiration, not as definitive course of action for any individual.

Preface

After going through Coronary Arterial Bypass Graph (CABG) surgery, I found it comforting to write down thoughts and memories in a small blank book as I recovered. These entries became a loose type of personal journal therapy. When I wrote a thought down, I was able to identify and let go of the potential emotional build-up connected to it. It helped me maintain proper focus on my physical recovery. It was a stress reliever, and it proved very effective.

Years later, as I sorted through and discarded cards and notes received after my surgery, I came across my little journal. As I read through the entries, they still had a calming and reassuring effect on me. I thought surely other heart patients would also benefit from these notes as I had. Hence, the idea for this book was birthed.

I put the book together as 50 short daily inspirational readings of encouragement. It begins with some of my thoughts and experiences just before and immediately following my own surgery and progresses to some of my present observations as a visitor of other heart patients years later. My hope is to accompany other heart patients, in the form of this easy-to-read book, through their recovery back to their own sense of normalcy. I chose the magic number of 50 readings because after 50 days, most heart patients have regained some semblance of a normal lifestyle.

I was initially going to name this book, *Give Yourself 50 Days*, because I am often asked how long it took to feel "normal" again. The short, over-simplified answer to that question is 6-8 weeks (50 days), but I felt the title settled on represents more of a companionship with the reader, with the intention of giving them a sense of being accompanied through their recovery. No one should ever go through anything like major surgery and recovery feeling like they are alone.

Lastly, I am a firm believer that whatever I may go through is not just for my own learning or benefit. If I can help others by sharing what I have gone through, it only gives my experience that much more meaning. Likewise, if I can learn from what others have gone through, I may also save myself some unnecessary hardship.

Diane Caputo

Contents

1. Having a Plan

How does one plan ahead for a heart "event"? Does any such plan exist? If it does, I didn't have one.

Most people go about their daily routines oblivious to their heart health. Whether we receive doctors' warnings of danger signs or purposely live an active, healthy lifestyle, our hearts involuntarily continue pumping. Some heart procedures are performed on patients after years of neglect or gradual decline in health. Sometimes they are thrust upon patients with little or no warning.

My heart event was totally unexpected; it was suddenly hurled upon my family and me. There were no warning signs. I didn't have a family history of heart disease. I didn't have high blood pressure or high cholesterol. I was not overweight and I maintained a healthy, active lifestyle. An undetected congenital problem in one of my arteries just showed its ugly face one day. When I was in the midst of my first attack, the words "heart attack" never entered my mind. In fact, I shrugged off my sudden symptoms of profuse sweat, nausea and weakness as having been caused by something bad I must have eaten the night before. It occurred first thing in the morning and felt like a bad case of morning sickness; but I knew *that* option for an explanation was not a possibility. The nausea passed quickly, in just a matter of a few minutes, and I resumed my daily routine without another thought about it. Everything seemed fine again.

I did not think about my heart until a second attack hit me three days later. This second attack fortunately had different symptoms than the first. This time I felt a heavy pressure bearing down on my chest pressing me into the couch on which I was sitting. It was unwilling to let me get up from the couch. This time I did think something was going on with my heart. I took two aspirins and two friends I call "my life savers" insisted on taking me to the nearest emergency room.

I know, I should have called 911, but it didn't occur to me that I was any kind of an emergency. Now I know.

Here's my point. Heart disease isn't anything one "plans" on having. If anything, we can try our best to be healthy enough to *prevent* it. One deals with heart disease after it "shows up," Our best plan of action is to diligently do what we know we should, and not do what we know we shouldn't, on a daily basis. All else is out of our control. Sometimes knowing what we should do and actually doing it can be two different things. It should include making oneself familiar with warning signs of heart trouble and the number to call in an emergency: 911. We can't plan a heart event, but we can know the right response if it shows its face anytime in the future.

2. No Unresolved Conflicts

My date with a heart surgeon came upon me with some degree of urgency. I was in the hospital Catherization (CATH) lab undergoing a relatively noninvasive procedure to insert a stent into my heart's trouble spot. Two stents later, they had not achieved their intended purpose, and my cardiologist informed me of my need for open heart surgery. My case was unusual. Most cases do not go to surgery directly from the CATH lab table, especially after receiving two stents. Most patients are given time of a day or so for recovery from the stent procedure before they are brought to open heart surgery, or, if surgery is needed, they may not insert stents at all.

My situation was termed "emergent." I took the announcement for surgery with remarkable calmness. I credit my ability to keep my composure to the grace of God upon me at that moment and the assumption I was already on some kind of "happy juice" helping me remain calm during the stent procedure. It was like I was being told I needed another minor procedure done in the next room. My head only registered, "No big deal," I waited in the CATH lab while my surgeon finished up on the patient ahead of me and prepared for his second major surgery of that day-mine.

Everyone in the lab wanted to keep me at ease while I laid there waiting; someone even retrieved a favorite CD from my belongings I had brought to the hospital. If you are familiar with the group 2nd

Chapter of Acts, the song "Sing Over Me" was proclaimed throughout the CATH lab as we all waited and listened. It continues to be a song of emotional comfort and reassurance to this day. My rings were then removed for surgery and delivered to my husband in the waiting room. A nurse asked me if there was anything else I desired. I asked if I could pray for the surgeon and his operating team. Some of the staff gathered around my bed and the only thing I specifically remember praying for was that no one would enter the operating room with any unresolved conflicts. I remember this probably because although it was a sincere, rational request on my part, it received a hardy chuckle from the surrounding staff. Apparently, they bore witness to it being a most appropriate request considering the surgical team. It was my last memory before surgery; I was then put to sleep at peace.

It was a couple days later when a nurse came into my room curious about meeting the gal who prayed for "no unresolved conflicts." He said he had heard a lot of prayers before surgery, usually for wisdom and guidance, but that request had been a first for him. I had a simple explanation. I needed everyone's heads to be clear and their minds sharp, especially for their second long surgery of the day. I figured the best way for that to happen would be for everyone present to be able to let go of anything else weighing on their minds, at least while operating on me! It was purely selfish on my part but an appropriate request just the same.

3. No Ring

Initially, I was only supposed to have a catherization procedure done to reopen a trouble spot in one of my arteries by inserting a stent. For this, I could remain awake and rings could stay on. I was able to view the monitors showing the stent insertion as the cardiologist did his work. Even I commented to him that blood didn't seem to be passing through that artery any better than before the stent was in place. He just glanced at me with no comment. Two stents later, it became clear I required bypass surgery. The cardiologist was clearly disappointed and apologetic.

Now all rings needed to be removed. It was the year of my 20th wedding anniversary. In all that time I never took my wedding ring off except to give it an occasional cleaning. I reluctantly removed it and handed it to my nurse as she promised to personally deliver it immediately to my husband out in the waiting room. I looked down at my hand as that funny little feeling remained on the empty finger reminding me something was definitely missing. It was a simple gold solitaire diamond ring, but it was *my* ring from the love of *my* life.

A few days later, I figured it was time to return my wedding ring to its proper place. Because I was still in the hospital, I asked my husband to bring my ring to me the next time he came from home. He got this awkward, twisted look on his face as he responded positively to my request. I interpreted that peculiar look as the expression of one who felt bad for not having thought of returning it to me already. I didn't want him to feel worse than he did; I dropped the subject. I was sure I would see my ring soon and return it to its proper place of residency.

The next day, to my disappointment, my husband did not produce the anticipated ring. He said something about bringing it had slipped his mind in the hustle of taking care of other pressing matters. Among other daily details, we had eight young children at home without their mother. There were plenty of other things vying for his attention.

I understood.

What no one else quite understood at this time, however, was that that little ring represented one of my steps back to a sense of normalcy in my life. I remained a bit emotionally disconnected as my ring remained disconnected from my finger.

To be continued...

4. The Waiting Room

The most anxious place during heart surgery is not necessarily the operating room. The waiting room can be a place of high anxiety for the patient's loved ones. Family and friends often gather together here for hours at a time awaiting word about the patient in surgery as they attempt to fill that time talking, sleeping, writing, or in other quiet activities. They are usually most appreciative of visitors who take the opportunity to reassure them that their loved one is in a highly reputable facility and is receiving the utmost care possible.

The patient at this time is oblivious to his situation. His (or her) need for encouragement and instruction is presently on hold. Doctors and medical staff generously share their knowledge and experience with the family in the waiting room. Thankfully, the staff is faithful to inform the family on the progress of their loved one's surgery as opportunity allows. They have studied their expertise and are highly skilled and passionate about what they do. I am glad there are people who know what they know; what an understatement! However, they have not experienced being the patient themselves. Even their experience is limited. Family members and friends, during this time, are often glad to receive a visit from someone who has personally been through the surgery. I receive the most questions about recovery, not from the patients, but from loved ones in the waiting room who are wondering what to expect in the next few hours, the next few days, and the next few weeks, etc. These people are not particularly going anywhere soon, so they usually appreciate passing some time having constructive conversation with someone who's been through the surgery. I'm not a medical expert; I'm just someone who understands pretty well what that patient is going to go through, both emotionally and physically, in the very near future. If I can take someone else's anxiety level down a notch or two, by sharing my own experience, it brings all the more understanding and purpose to the anxieties I and my family once went through.

5. What's That Noise?

As I lay in bed the night following my heart surgery, I slept off my anesthesia and experienced what I call a little "memory pocket." I recalled hearing the dull, somewhat distant, sound like that of a power saw. It was a little unnerving and two possible explanations immediately came to my mind simultaneously. The first was, "Wow, this hospital must be going through some renovations. What a crazy time of day for construction to be going on! I must be nearby where it is taking place."

My second thought was, "Hey, surgeons use saws to open patients' chests for operations! I must be near where a surgery is taking place. These walls don't muffle noise very well, because I would surely rather not hear that!" Before I could think much further on the subject, sleep once again overtook me, and cowardice restrained me from later finding out which possibility may have been the reality.

It was weeks later, as I was reviewing the journal I was keeping of my recovery, that the third possibility suddenly struck me. I may have actually experienced a "memory pocket" of the sound of my own surgery taking place! It was a little overwhelming at that moment to pursue that thought any further, so I closed my journal for reviewing another time. The first two possibilities instantly became equally preferred choices for the noise's origin.

Cowardice still keeps me from even wanting to know which, if any, of the three explanations is reality, or if the whole thing was just one of those weird post-operation dreams!
It's anyone's guess.

6. T is for Tongue

I laid in the Cardiac Intensive Care Unit (C.I.C.U) the night after my heart surgery for seemingly endless hours as I faded in and out of consciousness, dreaming off my anesthetics. I don't remember any tunnels of light or any beings beckoning me to stay. I had no grand dreams of being visited by loved ones who have passed away or of beautiful country sides, mountain streams, or exotic beaches. I felt like I was suspended in an endless fog, a limitless limbo. I do remember hearing one of my favorite voices, that of my husband, breaking through the fog, talking to one of my nurses.

My husband said, "I think she's waking up."

"Yes, I think so too," the nurse responded.

"Do you think she hears us?" my husband asked.

"Definitely," I thought to myself.

"Look, she's raising her hand," the nurse said.

"She's signing the letter T to us," my husband realized.

I wasn't completely conscious. I felt like my tongue was long, hard, and bulky. It was too cumbersome to be of any use in forming words. I couldn't convince my mouth to coordinate my lips and tongue together to speak so the best I could think of doing was to sign "T" for "Tongue" with my hand.

"Come on guys," I thought, "Do something about my hard tongue!"

They didn't understand.

I felt a tender kiss on my forehead from you know who, the love of my life, as I drifted back to sleep in frustration. I realized later the hard bulky thing in my mouth was my breathing tube still in place from my surgery. It was soon removed and the next time I woke up I discovered my tongue was fully operational.

7. The Hands

As I lay still on my back, feeling totally weak, groggy, and helpless after surgery, I guess I was a bit of a mess with dried blood and this funny blue color all over me. I wouldn't exactly know; I didn't see any of it, but my husband did. No one could have fully prepared him for his first glimpse of his wife after surgery. It didn't quite make sense when staff warned him that his wife would look like a cold, blue alien with assorted tubes protruding from various parts of her body. The first sight of a patient after surgery, I am told, is the most overwhelming. It gets better from there.

I distinctly remember a pair of compassionate hands as I dozed in the Cardiac Intensive Care Unit recovering after my heart surgery. These gentle hands began at my feet and worked their way upward to cleanse my skin back to its true color. I thought surely this was what it must be like to be visited by a minister of God. I was calmed by this simple gesture and encouraged that recuperation wouldn't be as tough as I once thought. I'll probably never know who that person was, but this is my best way of thanking them for their kindness.

When the hands were done, I had a huge ace bandage wrapped down the entire length of my left leg. That's the leg that offered up the "vein sacrifice" for my bypass surgery. That bandage also held in place drainage tubes coming from my chest cavity. I had three tubes draining my chest of any blood and fluids left inside from my operation.

Heart surgery patients keep these tubes in for a day to sometimes more than a week, as long as necessary. They are removed when their job is done. Sometimes, the sooner they are removed, the sooner a patient can be discharged from the hospital. Mine remained in place doing their function for the next three days. This is pretty normal. One great benefit of getting these tubes removed is that the first post operation shower can then be taken. Everything about recovery seems a little more bearable after the tubes are removed and one has that first shower.

8. Glorious Ice Chips

One seemingly insignificant detail of my first night after heart surgery was the ice chips. I'm convinced no one could possibly understand or relate to what I mean unless they too have had major surgery. When I was waking up coming off the anesthesia, it was like my body's reset button had been pushed. Every part of my body was turning on again. As I began to eat again, it was like I was tasting everything I was given for the first time.

All night long, a nurse seemed to come by quite often to scan me over for inspection. On one such occasion she asked me if I would like some ice chips. I replied yes and a teaspoon of them was brought to my lips. I thought they were the most wonderful ice chips in the world! I was completely in the present-just me and those ice chips. I desired nothing else at that moment. How could something so simple be so satisfying? I was ready and willing, from that time forward, to spend the rest of my life sucking solely on ice chips one teaspoon at a time. My thoughts were totally consumed with nothing but glorious ice chips. If only I could remain so thankful all the time, but life obviously isn't that simple, or "glorious."

Morning would surely come with a new set of challenges beyond sucking ice chips.

9. Who Put the Board in My Chest?

The morning after my surgery arrived and so did the requirements. My chest felt as though it had been opened up, a 2x4 board was placed inside vertically, and then closed back up again. Not only that, but the "board" was pressing down on my chest. Don't forget I had three chest drainage tubes sticking out of my diaphragm too, which have already been mentioned. I was only able to take the shallowest of breaths as I could not adequately expand my chest. I felt I was barely bringing in enough oxygen to live. I had oxygen entering in through my nose, (yes another tube), and was convinced I would not survive without it. I discovered breathing from my diaphragm helped, a little.

That was about the time my nurse came by and informed me she was going to remove my oxygen tube.

"Are you sure?" I asked pitifully, "I feel like I'm hardly breathing."

She reassured me saying, "Your oxygen saturation in your blood is good. Besides, your oxygen tube has been shut off for hours already! You're doing fine."

I thought to myself, "This is surely the beginning of a string of lessons I am about to learn from a source outside my own understanding." I was going to have to trust something and/or someone beyond my finite perspective. In my case, that outside source definitely included the hospital nursing staff.

My breaths were short, shallow, and uncomfortable. I asked the nurse, "When will it get easier to breathe?"

She answered, "Tomorrow, it will be much easier."

"Tomorrow," I thought, as I immediately turned to look at the big, round, institutional clock on the wall. It read 11:30 A.M., and I said to myself, "I'm counting on today's grace to get me to tomorrow."

I watched the clock slowly tick as I practiced my breathing, repeating over and over, "Tomorrow."

"Tomorrow."

10. The Pillow

I was presented "the pillow" the morning after my heart surgery. Mine is heart shaped with a red floral pattern on it. At my hospital alone, thousands of these pillows have been given to heart patients over the years by a volunteer group called "The Needlers." Their special identification label is stitched onto every pillow they make. These volunteers are invisible except for their pillows. They and their pillows are one of the hospital's hidden gems. I've never seen or met a Needler that I know of, but each heart patient receives one of their pillows and is instructed not to keep it more than an arm's length away. It's kept nearby for immediate access and use.

Every pillow is appropriately heart-shaped and each is made of a different material making them unique for each patient. I soon learned it served a very important function. The nurse laid mine near my chest and instructed me that if I needed to cough, sneeze, or move my chest in any way, I was to hug it firmly in front of myself with my two arms crossed over it. It was there to help hold my freshly stitched chest secure.

The pillow has been a faithful companion; it brought me through many an anxious cough or sneeze. It accompanied me through my recuperation. To this day it receives a place of distinction in the pile of pillows that daily sit on top of my bed.

11. 30 Long Minutes

As I lay on my back the morning after my heart surgery, a nurse came in and informed me I was ready to sit up in a chair for 30 minutes. I couldn't believe such an otherwise simple task could be required of me so soon. I was in no position to argue. I was like a helpless child receiving instruction. I had to comply. Two nurses, one on each side of me, helped me sit up and held me steady. Immediately, I was nauseous and I began to heave. Fortunately, I had not eaten since before my surgery so there was nothing in my stomach (except for those glorious ice chips).

I quickly grabbed my heart pillow to ease the pressure I felt against my sutures which were getting a good joggling. My only thought was to calm the nausea as soon as possible.

After an eternal minute or two, the nausea passed. Nausea avoidance now became my primary goal in life, but, alas, I was merely upright in my bed. I was still short of the goal. Those nurses wanted me sitting in a chair. After one more nauseous heave, I was there. The nurses propped me up and secured me into a wheelchair by packing pillows between me and the chair. Then they left. They just left me there, stuffed in position. While I did my time in the chair, they tended to their other business. Obviously, I was not the only patient in that busy hospital. Others needed assistance. As I sat like a blob, my foggy brain could only wonder how my next transition back from chair to bed would go.

As I passed the time, an x-ray technician came in with a portable x-ray machine. He jammed an x-ray plate behind my back, took a picture, and off he went. What a guy. He definitely didn't make the same compassionate impression the "hands" did.

When my 30 minutes were up, nurses reappeared and I was gently guided back up to my bed. Oh, the thankfulness one can have for the slightest comfort. The nausea was gone. I didn't heave, choke, or cough unless I specifically willed to do so. What a relief to regain the slightest control over my own body.

12. Pastoral Care

A woman minister came to visit me as I lay in the Cardiac I.C.U. the morning after my surgery. I think I was placed on her list of routine rounds she took each day. Her voice was gentle, and her introduction was obviously rehearsed many times before. Her name flew by my hazy brain uncaught. I did hear her ask me if I would like to pray with her. "Oh yes," I said, as I reached for her hand.

I thanked God for another day and then for His grace to face it. I thanked Him for friends, family, surgeons, and staff, as the faces of those people flashed before my mind's eye. I thanked Him for the wisdom He places in men that His glory may be revealed in all circumstances.

As I finished, I glanced up at the minister who paused and looked straight at me for a moment. I then realized she had expected to do the praying. She seemingly re-gathered her own thoughts and added a prayer on my behalf for a quick and complete recovery.

"Oh yes," I said again, realizing I had forgotten to pray for my own healing. "That would be great. Thank you."

We said an "amen" together, and with a kind smile she turned to leave. As she left, I could not help but wonder if she enjoyed her vocation, and about the large range of responses she must get as she visited diverse people each day.

13. For the T Shirt

The day after my heart surgery, my nurse dutifully informed me that I would be moving to the 11th floor of the hospital for further recuperation. This all sounded fine and dandy until she told me I was to walk out of the C.I.C.U. myself and then they would take me the rest of the way to my new room in a wheelchair.

"Oh my," I said, "are you sure I can do that?"

She had confidence written all over her face as she responded, "The seventy-nine-year-old gentleman who had open heart surgery before you walked 30 paces to the double door exit out of here, I'm sure you can do it too."

I had to do it. It became a matter of determination and pride. After all, if someone almost twice my age could do it, so could I. So, with my husband beside me for my first steps, I eased myself up and steadied myself while holding on to the hand grips on the back of a wheelchair. My eyes and concentration were fixed on the double doors as I shuffled my slippered feet toward them.

The nurse chimed in again saying, "You know, you only get the T-shirt if you make it to the double doors."

I thought, "She can't be serious. I'm concentrating here. That is not a funny joke."

Well, I made it to the doors and was gently guided into the seat of the wheelchair I was pushing. I had earned passage to my new room out of Cardiac I.C.U. and on to 11th floor recovery.

Chalk up one small victory on the road of my recovery.

It turned out the nurse was serious about the T-shirt. Before I was discharged a few days later, I was presented a T-shirt which read, "I walked out of CICU." My hospital tries to give those T-shirts to all their patients who walk out those double doors.

14. Thanks to Real People

Heart surgery has a way of forcing us, in some way, to face our own mortality. I think it has something to do with the inescapable fact that no one lives without a heart. So when something goes wrong with it, we are brought to a place, sooner or later, of realizing how fragile our lives are. This can be a good learning time if dealt with in the right way.

When I found myself in my hospital room one day leaning this way in my thoughts, it wasn't great plans or unfinished tasks that filled my mind. It was people, loved ones, who struck my heart to continue its beating. People, those beings large and small, young and old, who hassle us, interrupt us, and manipulate us on a daily basis. They are a huge source from which I realize my true worth.

That all said, I'd like to recall and thank a few of those people that surrounded me through my recovery and continue to encourage me on my ongoing journey. We are all surrounded by such people and have the capability of being such a person. We sometimes just need our eyes opened to it.

To the friends and family who were instantly present…

To those who were compelled to pray…

To those who thought to call, and did…

To those who had to give the news we didn't want to hear…

To those who delivered words of good news and hope...

To those with that look of understanding when no words were transpired...

To those who shared words that broke through our emotions...

To all my caregivers with a gentle touch and those with a firm hand...

Thank you.

15. Questions Are Good

When someone goes through heart surgery, before they leave the hospital, they are usually given an overload of information about their procedure, recovery, and possible lifestyle changes. It may take some time and thought after surgery before the patient has a chance to formulate any questions or concerns for themselves. Sooner or later, though, questions will arise. How far should I be walking? How much rest is appropriate? When can I drive? What are possible side effects to my new medications? When should I go to rehabilitation classes? When can I take that trip I was planning? When will my appetite return? Once the questions start coming, the answers often lead to more questions.

Sometimes the patient feels they are being burdensome to their caregivers or medical staff with their questions. This couldn't be further from the truth. Questions are always good. They assist everyone, not just the patient, in dealing with the anxieties and individual circumstances surrounding each procedure. It's also good to ask until the answer is fully comprehended. This may not happen the first time a question is asked. Everyone has different degrees of knowledge about their own body and procedure. Ask until you are convinced your concerns have been addressed to the best capability. As one of my grade school teachers once said, "When one person asks a question, it often means several others had the same question, but didn't ask." Ask boldly; questions often help more people than just the one doing the asking.

16. What Happened to My Appetite?

The morning after my surgery, I needed to sit up for a little while without being nauseous. Then I was allowed to eat. My first meal after surgery was hot cereal. I'm not exactly a hot cereal kind of eater, but it tasted great to me. I was hungry, but I needed to start eating again slowly. I was told not to be surprised if I lost my appetite and up to 10 pounds during my initial recovery. Well, that was not the case with me. It wasn't long before I was hungry for more. Looking back, I seemed ravenous. I was always looking forward to my next meal, and everything tasted great. I had no complaints about the "institutional" hospital food.

Not everyone is like this. I hear story after story of people who wake up after their surgery having lost their appetites. This is very common. Nothing sounds appetizing; nothing tastes good. Of course, hospital food isn't known to be gourmet, but they do a good job serving up some heart-healthy meal options. Many patients have to be encouraged to eat in order to regain their strength. In fact, if the patient doesn't eat, they will be warned they may have to be fed intravenously. The idea after surgery is to get rid of tubes coming from one's body, not to keep them in!

Most people regain their appetite after a few days or so as their body's systems all wake up and get back to working properly. Surprisingly, I know of one case in which the patient never regained his appetite. It's been years since his surgery, and this patient still has to remind himself to eat each day. It has definitely contributed to his weight loss program. He has lost over 80 pounds and says he feels better than he did 30 years ago. He's learned that if he's feeling a little light-headed in the afternoon, he probably hasn't eaten and he'd better feed himself soon. He has had to adjust his lifestyle to eating without feeling hunger in order to maintain his health.

I know; all you readers are wishing if only you could have the same problem! However, he maintains it's not as wonderful as it sounds. He has had to learn to eat even when his body doesn't tell him to, and he doesn't always remember to do so, especially when he's by himself. We don't realize what a gift a thing like hunger can be.

17. The First Sneeze

Heart surgery recovery moves forward by a series of small victories. Somewhere along this road, the intersection of the first sneeze is crossed. I did not think about sneezing until I felt the first one rising up within me. It suddenly became one of those otherwise commonplace occurrences to be avoided by any means.

I distinctly remember that heightened breath one feels just before a sneeze. I was only a few days out from my surgery in my hospital room bed. I grabbed my heart pillow, placed it in position over my chest, and braced myself for the coming explosion. With my eyes wide open, a vision flew across my mind of each staple and stitch blowing out across the room. My husband saw the concern on my face and froze in position next to me, watching. Time stopped for an instant. Then, as quickly as it came upon me, the sneeze disintegrated into a huge exhalation. We both let out a deep sigh of relief. The sneeze's time had not yet come.

I had one more false sneeze alarm about a week or so after the first with much less drama. My personal first sneeze victory did not come that day either.

I had a good friend, Bob, who had heart surgery a couple years before me. He remembered the anxiety and discomfort he felt as he experienced his first "post-surgery sneeze." Unbeknownst to me, he had decided his personal prayer would be for me to make it through my initial days of recovery without having to sneeze.

My first sneeze did come, and I made it through just fine with very little drama. Everything stayed in place! It was another small victory. Even a few weeks out from surgery, the first sneeze was a little unnerving, but my pillow was braced in place. I knew I'd be fine. All sneezes thereafter were a "breeze."

Answered prayer? Decide for yourself, but I'll thankfully take it. Weakness has a way of bringing us to a place of receiving help in lots of forms, from lots of sources.

Bob has since passed away and gone to where there is no more heart disease, but his legacy of prayer for the prolonged avoidance of the first sneeze continues on after him.

18. Daily Diligence

My date with heart surgery came suddenly, without warning time to line up child care for my eight children. Shortly after my admittance to the hospital, our newlywed neighbors immediately came to our house freeing my husband to be by my bedside. They virtually moved into our home to care for our children and called it a privilege. Wow!

From my hospital room, I often inquired how my neighbor was faring in my busy home. I only got the report that she loved the opportunity to give, and called my household a "well-oiled machine." My first response to that was, "Is she in MY house?" Everyone must have been on their best behavior. I was relieved.

I was so thankful for the little organizational details our family practiced each day, the repetitive things I continually reminded our children. You know the ones; they are the daily tasks we wonder whether they will ever remember to do without being told, like brushing their teeth, making beds, picking up socks, taking out the trash, saying please and thank you. These everyday lessons rehearsed and repeated over and over again in ordinary day-to-day life can pay off in unexpected times.

I say all this as a reminder for us all not to despise our own personal daily vocations. What we do on a daily basis has payoffs we may not immediately witness. One practical bit of advice given to me that I wish to pass on to other patients I visit is, "Don't get ahead of yourself. Face one day at a time. Be present. Where are you, what are you doing, and who are you with? That's exactly where you should be." Your daily diligence will have its rewards, in its perfect time, possibly when you least expect it.

19. How About Those Nurses?

While I was recovering in the hospital, several nurses made an unforgettable impression upon me. Don't expect names here; just fill in your nurse's name if the shoe fits. Are there people out there that choose the nursing profession because of the incredibly fantastic salary? I stand by a pretty strong conviction that the majority of nurses are such because somehow, they felt a "calling" to it. These nurses love their vocation because it's about the people, not just the job. The kind of compassion and attention to detail they must exhibit on a daily basis isn't entirely learned in a classroom or text book.

One nurse in particular would stop by my room to check in with me even when it was clear she did not have to. I noticed. It is such a treat to witness someone who has a passion for what they do… especially when I receive the benefit! It's those seemingly insignificant gestures, that may pass unnoticed, that make the difference.

Another nurse knew just what to say in order to boost my confidence and recuperation to the next level. This nurse always knew what I was capable of doing before I did. With guiding hands and encouraging speech, they were always able to convince me of performing that next step in my recovery.

I met up with one nurse weeks after my release from the hospital, and she asked me how everything was going. I replied, "It's going as well as can be expected."

The nurse responded, "You are one of the reasons I do what I do. Seeing people get better makes it all worth it."

So here's to you nurses, and anyone else, who say, through your acts of both duty and compassion, "Fulfillment in our lives comes as a result of our outward acts toward others."

20. Doing Nothing

When I came home from the hospital after my surgery, I was instructed to do "nothing" for 3 weeks. For someone recovering from heart surgery, this doesn't technically mean do nothing. It means you are allowed to push, pull, or lift only if you experience no pain when you do so. I was told not to let anything I carry weigh more than a gallon of milk. I personally recommend refraining from housework and driving for this time period if that's possible. These instructions are meant to protect the chest incision and allow it time to heal properly. Overdoing anything involving the chest muscles could lead to prolonging one's recovery, or worse, to infection that may land the patient back in the hospital.

My legs worked fine, so I could go for walks, but I was to split up those walks with plenty of rest. I could gradually extend the length of my walk each time. Our bodies do their best healing while we are at rest and sleeping, so alternating resting and walking proves to be the best plan of action. Years ago, if someone had heart surgery, the patient was assigned to bed rest for weeks afterward. This is definitely no longer the norm. Patients are gotten up and encouraged to walk as soon as they are able, often before they know they are able, as in my case. It amazed me how soon my heart was ready to do its work. Today, the mentality behind heart surgery recovery is to get the heart doing what it was created to do as soon as possible-pumping and circulating blood.

I thought about all the reading I was going to catch up on while I rested. I didn't realize that my concentration levels would be a bit wacky for some time after surgery, so I wasn't able to read and retain as much as I would have liked. It was a minor detail that only I really noticed about myself. No one informed me about this little side effect of surgery, but after talking to many other patients, I find it is a common experience. So, think it not strange if you are reading along and you suddenly stop and say to yourself, "What did I just read?" This too will pass. Okay, it still happens to me on occasion, but I think that is normal for everyone! Keep on reading. You will gradually realize your concentration level has returned.

21. Sleeping Inclined

I was fortunate to have a hospital bed awaiting me when I came home from the hospital. (I never realized how heavy one of those things is.) A group of strong friends got it for me and set it up in our main floor guest bedroom. It was kind of fun, initially, playing around with the settings in order to find my most comfortable position. Many patients who don't have access to a hospital bed find using a recliner chair very helpful for the same purpose of resting inclined for some time after surgery. I preferred keeping the head of the bed raised for a couple very practical reasons. For one, getting in and out of bed was much easier with it in an inclined position. I could just throw my legs off the side of the bed and then roll the rest of me out to follow them. This practically helped keep the need to use my upper body muscles down to a minimum.

Secondly, I found it a bit unnerving to lay flat for quite some time after my surgery. Whenever I would lay flat I became overly aware of my beating heart. I just wanted to know it was beating; I didn't necessarily want to hear each beat and feel each thump. If I kept the head of the bed raised, the inside of my chest seemed quieter, and I was able to rest peacefully.

As the weeks of my recovery passed, I gradually lowered the incline of the bed until it was flat again. My transitions in and out of bed became easier and easier. It eventually became clear the time had come to return to my own bed in my own bedroom.

It was one more small victory toward my goal back to normal daily life.

22. Getting Cozy

When I was released from the hospital after surgery, I was cleared to do two things: walk and rest, with emphasis on the rest. Normally in my household, during the day, I am the chief motivator, delegator, and servant. Running a large household requires the continual performance of lots of small tasks. I suddenly needed many forms of help. Some tasks had to be put on hold while others were done differently than I was used to having them done. Does anyone know how hard that can be for a mother who is used to continually having something to do, to be slowed down into the role of chief observer and receiver of assistance?

After a couple days of this, everyone (everyone meaning my 8 children) around me was "resting" also. They were merely following my lead. They were enjoying the new restful atmosphere of our home. It was like my household entered perpetual weekend relaxation mode, but, as everyone else got more and more cozy, I got more and more restless. Other mothers, I'm sure, understand what I'm talking about. In a household of 10 people like mine, it doesn't take long for entropy to set in; things were naturally flowing from order to disorder. I started seeing undone tasks all around me, and I imagined other tasks that I couldn't directly see. I did what any other sane mother would do; I began pointing to children and assigning jobs. I exclaimed, "If Momma aint at rest, aint nobody at rest." I would rest well once order was reestablished. I would continue to rest as order was maintained.

Since everyone wanted Mom resting and recuperating, everyone got moving again to do their part in keeping order (and peace) in the home. I, sporting a playful smile, assured my children they need not worry. I would let them know, though highly unlikely, if they were found over exerting themselves. No child labor laws were violated. It was a simple plan with simple execution, both needing a necessary sense of humor at all times.

23. Tingling Fingers and Toes

No one has ever shared a similar experience to this with me, but if I share it here, someone may recall their own experience with it.

As I was recovering at home from my surgery, I sometimes woke up from a nap, and my fingertips and/or my toes would be numb. I would also wake up this way during the night. After a few shakes or wiggles, they would regain feeling and I would be fine, but, since it would happen with some regularity, it was a little unsettling. After all, numbness refers to lack of circulation, and circulation refers to the heart, and MY heart was the thing that was supposed to be repaired. I placed "numbness in my fingertips" at the top of my list of questions for my follow-up appointment with my cardiologist.

When I asked my cardiologist about it, I was glad to hear he was unalarmed. His calm response eased my concern. He said to just wiggle the toes or shake out the fingers like I had been doing and the symptoms would eventually go away. For months it seemed finger shaking would be part of my regular routine. I got used to it. Then, as time passed, I shook them less and less often. One day, about six months after my surgery, I realized I had not performed my shake-and-go routine for quite some time. The symptom had faded so gradually, I wasn't sure exactly when it had stopped. So, always check in with medical staff concerning symptoms, but don't be too alarmed that some may persist longer than expected.

24. Skip the Gory Details

For weeks after my surgery, friends would come by with dinners and to inquire how my recovery was coming along. On one such occasion, friends were asking about some of the details of my recent heart history. As I described some of the circumstances leading up to and including my bypass surgery, I began to get a little emotional. Tears began to well up in my eyes. Memories were still a little too fresh. Well, a hot dinner was on the table; we were all hungry, but I did not want to appear ungrateful to our generous friends by quickly sending them on their way.

One of our daughters observed my failing attempt to make a long story short and came to my defense. She knew some of my details were just too much for me to bear so soon. I needed rescuing. She interrupted with such clear spontaneity that everyone gladly turned, in unison, to give her their attention.

She announced, "Basically, the doctors had to go in and fix the 'ucky' in my Mom's heart. Now she has shiny fresh blood properly flowing through it." We all smiled at one another as we all agreed that was about all we needed to know. "Ucky" covered a lot of ground and spared a lot of words; the rest was just gory detail.

I'm thankful for the simplicity of children.

25. The Secret Handshake

Once I was discharged from the hospital, friends would stop by and visit me at my home. I love visitors. Two dear friends came by one day with a wonderful chicken dinner for our family.

(Just a side note here: Bringing dinner to my household is no small endeavor. Anyone bringing dinner to my hungry family with eight children must surely be committed to us! Dinner is no small act of charity!)

Anyway, one of these friends, Bob, previously had heart surgery like mine. We were both recipients of a triple bypass. We declared ourselves members of the fictitious "Tri-By" club. We are not offended by anyone who does not want to go through what it takes to become a member of our club, that's for sure.

Bob showed me the "secret" handshake of our club. Can you imagine what it would be? He clasped my hands and then gently squeezed and released two times in a row and paused. He then squeezed gently again two more times and released my hands. He was imitating the beat of our hearts in the handshake.

We both had a great hardy laugh together. I guess having heart surgery can give one some new perspectives on humor.

So if you have had, or meet someone who has had, heart surgery, go ahead; share the handshake and share a smile.

26. Cardiac Rehabilitation

A couple days after being released from the hospital following my bypass surgery, someone from my hospital's cardiac rehabilitation program called me at home and scheduled me to begin classes with them. The very next week I began a 16 session program, two days a week, over the next eight weeks. Just as a side note, I hear insurance companies cover the expense of more sessions now for patients who desire to attend rehabilitation classes. That tells me how important it must be to both cardiologists and insurance companies for qualifying patients to participate.

To say I was nervous on my first day is an understatement. As far as I was concerned, my body had betrayed me and a working relationship between me and it was going to have to be reestablished. Some kind of trust level had to be rebuilt. I was extremely reluctant to ask my body to perform any physical exertion.

I walked into the classroom and was immediately surprised at the number of people in there. I was in my early forties; most of the other participants were old enough to be my parents. Seems the average age for heart surgery is somewhere around seventy. Someone my age is a bit less common. One person sitting next to me asked if I had accompanied one of my parents to the class. No, I had to admit, I qualified to be there because I myself had surgery. Several people immediately took it upon themselves to look out for the "youngster."

Every class begins by having each person's blood pressure and weight recorded. Then a portable EKG is hooked up to monitor each participant's heart. After about a half hour class covering heart related subjects such as diet and medications, everyone heads out to the exercise room.

As I walked what seemed like baby steps around the perimeter of the room, I cautiously eyeballed my corresponding EKG monitor display along the side of the room. Amazingly, it remained absolutely normal with every lap I took. Apparently, I was going to survive my first physical exertion.

I enjoyed talking to the people there. There was no evidence of anger and/or self-pity. In fact, there was a spirit of thankfulness for being "still here." I gained as much confidence from hearing of other patient's recoveries as I did from participating in the physical rehabilitation. I called them my little "preordained visits of personal encouragement." Cardiac rehabilitation participation became the single most important recommendation I would give to other recovering heart patients from then on.

27. The Fading Scar

As I recuperated from heart surgery, I wanted to know how to properly take care of my scars. My scarlet colored chest scar was very conspicuous against the rest of my fair skin. I felt like people saw the scar when they looked at me, instead of my face. The less attention drawn to it, the better. I was willing to do whatever I could to help it heal well and blend in with my surrounding skin. People gave me various tips like rubbing vitamin E onto the scar and keeping sun block and clothing over it to prevent the sun from hitting it. All this I did willingly and diligently. Everyone assured me the crimson scar would fade; they said to give it time. I wanted to know how much time it would take.

As I participated in cardiac rehabilitation, it was one of my initial questions for the group. Many people had various answers to the question. Some had scars that faded rather quickly, within a few months after their surgery. Others said it took much longer to fade. Mine easily took over a year to settle on its final shade. So, I guess the answer is to be patient, it will fade. It takes as long as it takes. Ten years later, I hardly notice my scar, and neither does anyone else. But when I do look at it, I am reminded how my heart surgery has become a part of my life story. It has played a part in forming me into who and where I am now, alive and well.

28. Return to Me

There's a great movie called *Return to Me*. It's about a heart transplant recipient, named Grace, played by Minnie Driver. It's full of colorful friends and family and I always have fun envisioning my own dear friends and family members inserted into the characters throughout the movie.

There is a great scene in the movie in which Grace is in the midst of revealing an emotionally distressing secret she's been bearing alone to her close friend Megan. Megan's husband walks in on the conversation and sees them both crying. He quickly perceives something serious is going on. He starts guessing what it is and comes to all the wrong assumptions. The emotions between the three of them escalate until the big secret is finally blurted out. The air immediately clears as the declaration shocks everyone back into their right minds once again and life moves on.

I say all this to remind heart patients that stress during recovery can get overwhelming at times. Sometimes emotions can pop out with seemingly no prompting. One minute everything is fine; the next minute unexplainable tears may be falling. This is not uncommon in the heart patient. Part of a healthy healing process is to have friends or family around with whom we can share and release any anxieties we face. Friends always want to know how they can help during someone else's recovery. One huge way our friends and caregivers practically give to us is by listening. It seems insignificant but it is not. Talking helps relieve emotional buildup. If we take care of thoughts and cares as they come up, hopefully an emotional explosion can be avoided.

29. Thankfulness vs. Depression

After heart surgery, I experienced two opposite emotional poles. Like the swing of a pendulum, there were two extremes and an infinite number of intermediate variations in between. They were like two hidden forces vying for my attention.

On one side of the pendulum was great thankfulness for the opportunity to experience another day in my seemingly insignificant life. Here I found myself inspired by every conversation and interaction. Nothing was trivial. I wanted to listen to others and also to testify of my own thankfulness. My conversations seemed to get more candid. Everyone I knew suddenly became more precious. I felt more "present" in my current circumstances. Simple things in life became hugely significant. I was glad to merely open my eyes and face each new day. This sense of well-being can't be mustered up by sheer will. It's a remarkably positive after-effect of such a serious surgery.

The other extreme side of the pendulum struck much less often as an inexplicable heaviness of worthlessness that would surge over me like a sudden wave. Sometimes unprompted, unexplainable tears would appear trickling down my cheeks. This side of the swing would usually reveal itself in the dark quiet of night or when I was alone and most vulnerable to discouraging thoughts which were usually not even founded in truth. It always attempted to keep me alone in my thoughts, both mentally and physically, and to keep me from admitting to the emotional attack.

My immediate defense is a spoken proclamation. Rattling off the many people and circumstances I am thankful for issues back in a sense of peace to my inner spirit. Another reality to replace the current false downtrodden situation must be immediately constructed. Doing this before real live people whenever possible is most ideal. There is always strength in numbers, but, I am ultimately the one responsible for where I allow my own thoughts to go. My mind becomes a battleground over what is going to rule my thoughts, and I am the commander in chief fighting it.

I'm not sure why these two battling emotions seem to accompany heart surgery recovery. It's too common to deny. Think it not strange when the battle arises. Many find consolation knowing they are not alone in the experience. Obviously, everyone welcomes the positive side of the emotional swing. Conversely, realizing the negative emotional swing can take place in each of us also holds the key to the victory through it. Get a friend, a sibling, a support group, and enter the good fight to keep yourself in your right mind.

30. Scar Shame

I was initially self-conscious about my chest scar. I felt like a reluctant walking billboard for heart surgery. It was the last thing I wanted to advertise. At my age, especially, I didn't like people knowing I had a heart condition. (Okay, I was 42 at the time; now you know) I preferred not to draw any attention to that fact if I could help it. Neck lines went up. Necklaces got bulky. I kept my scar covered and out of sight for the most part.

Then, one day at the bank, the teller happened to notice my scar. She too had had heart surgery revealed a scar similar to mine. We connected instantly in conversation. We understood what the other had been through, both emotionally and physically. A sense of strength and inspiration was exchanged.

That conversation marked the end of scar hiding. My thinking took a one-hundred-eighty-degree turn. Now I wear my scar shamelessly. If seeing my scar initiates a conversation with someone, and we're able to exchange some moments of hope and encouragement, I welcome it. Because of a scar, I have engaged in many conversations of hope that may never have happened otherwise. Doing so gives me great satisfaction. My experience of weakness has become a means to strengthen others. What we go through in life isn't only for our own learning and growth. As we grow through what we learn and experience, we have the potential to multiply it by each person to whom we pass along that learning.

31. No Ring (continued)

I had taken off my wedding ring because of my need to have surgery. My last recollection was that it dwelled safely in my husband's possession. Days later, I was ready to ditch the hospital gown, put on some *real* clothes, and be discharged from the hospital. My outfit would be complete once my ring was returned to my finger.

My husband arrived to take me home, but he still did not produce a ring for my finger. This day, he told me he must have misplaced it in the pocket of his pants he wore the week before. I knew I was helpless with that answer. I had not been home to sort through his laundry to catch a passing ring. I began to be concerned, but my husband remained confident that it would show up if he back tracked and checked his most recently worn pants' pockets. I remained calm.

The subject of the missing ring was never brought up unless I brought it up. I joggled between not wanting to pressure my husband about finding it and being upset that no one except for me seemed to be concerned about finding it. Another week or so passed, and by then I had formed my own search and rescue effort. I sought out every pair of my husband's pants and checked every pocket-no ring. I even searched every square inch of my house with the same result. Yes, I strategically did this without performing any heavy pushing or pulling! My face could no longer hide signs of despair.

My husband approached me, with an uneasy smile, holding a ring. Finally, I thought. To my disappointment, it was only my wedding band. Well, I told myself, at least it was something. I put it back on my finger as he confessed the simple gold band was all he was able to find. My spirit sank. He suggested taking apart the washer and/or dryer to see if it had possibly fallen down inside either of them. He promised he would do this the next chance he got. My hope was rekindled. Still, I was beginning to tell myself my diamond may never be seen again. It was time to make a choice.

I chose to be thankful for the *many* things I possessed and not to be upset about the *one* thing I no longer possessed. Some situations can't be controlled, but I can control how I respond to them. To be continued...

32. 4 Weeks and Counting

Four weeks after my surgery, I was still adjusting to the reality of everything I had been through since that day. I was stronger each day, and many of my daily tasks had been resumed. Some days I woke up and my first thoughts were as everything was before my operation. I momentarily felt as if my surgery and recuperation up to that point were just part of the previous night's dreams. It took a few moments for reality to kick in. I figured as I slept, my brain was still sorting, filtering and filing the emotional and physical information it had recently received. So it was easy to believe all was as it once was, until I moved, of course.

Other days, I woke up overwhelmingly thankful I literally woke up! I found myself wanting to talk with and listen to everyone I saw. I guess my eyes had been opened a bit to how fragile life can be and how petty we can be with so many details of it.

One big lesson I'm beginning to understand is that my whole experience with my heart event isn't a "set back" to get through or to put behind me somehow and try to forget. It's become part of the entire journey that's constantly forming me into who I am. Through the help of suffering (yes, suffering) and friends, I can choose to "look at the bright side" so to speak. I've been able to put a good construction on a seemingly not-so-good situation. Somehow, this extends to every person with whom I come in contact and with whom I have some level of relationship. I desire to pass on the hope I've received and multiply it through sharing it with others.

I believe this is a piece of what is meant in Romans 5:3-5 where it says, "...we glory in tribulations also: knowing that tribulation works patience; and patience, experience; and experience, hope: and hope makes us not ashamed..." Go ahead, ask me about my surgery, recovery, or ongoing lifestyle; I'm not ashamed.

33. Hearts are Created to Pump

The human heart is an amazing organ. From the moment it begins to beat, long before we are born, until our death, it continuously pumps our blood. Okay, I understand those who have had the glorious privilege of temporarily being on a heart lung machine have experienced a slight interruption of this process. Our heart is an involuntary muscle; it does its job, whether we're awake or asleep, without us consciously willing it to do so. I have read that for an average lifespan of seventy-five years at a pace of seventy beats per minute, the human heart will beat about 2.75 billion times. Now that is an efficient piece of work!

Following my surgery, I was initially afraid to require anything beyond resting state from my heart. I didn't want to make it do anything it no longer was capable of or willing to do. Cardiac Rehabilitation helped immensely in reestablishing a working relationship between my heart and the rest of my body. It sounds elementary, but during my rehabilitation, one thing I had to relearn was that my heart was a muscle, and muscles are created to work. A working muscle is a healthy, happy muscle. Bringing our heart rate up, through cardio aerobic exercise, is good maintenance for it. Interval training type exercise is also quite good for our hearts. This is when exercise is done in such a way as to alternate between bringing the heart rate up and down throughout the exercise session. The benefits of a morning workout actually extend out through the day. Attention levels are said to be improved after exercise, and many report to be less tired during the day. Exercise is actually a huge key to prolonging the lifespan of one's heart. The old expression "Use it, or lose it" definitely applies to our muscles, including our heart.

So keep the heart healthy by exercising it and giving it good nutrition. Even our rest times are proven to be more restful when we take part in a regular aerobic exercise program. It makes sense to help the heart, in any way we can, do what it was created to do.

34. Plateaus in Recovery

Recovery from heart surgery plays out like a series of baby steps, or what I like calling them-little victories. Getting the breathing tube out upon regaining consciousness is one of the first victories. Taking steps and extending the distance gone on each walking effort are more victories. Being discharged from the hospital is yet another victory, and on it goes until the patient has arrived back to a sense of well-being and normalcy in their life.

Many patients move steadily along their course of recovery with very few bumps. Mine happened to be like that. Conversely, others experience times when their recovery seems to reach a plateau. These are pockets of time when it seems recovery is at a standstill somewhere less than the goal the patient has set for himself. It's easy for discouragement to take hold here. Patients may begin to believe this is the condition they have to settle on for the rest of their lives. Of course, many physical explanations can be behind this experience. Understandably, everyone has his own set of extenuating circumstances that must be taken into consideration here.

Not so fast. There's a huge point to make here. Be encouraged; continue the rehabilitation. Faithfully do what you can; stay the course. Your body is going through a huge healing process. Give it some understanding. It always helps to know you're not alone in this experience. Experiencing plateaus is probably more often the case than not, and they can occur at any point in the recovery, but those that press on most often find the plateaus are temporary. The dips in the road are part of the path. This is one of those times when audible encouragement plays a huge role. Sometimes that "outside" word from someone else like a friend carries strength in it that we don't have for ourselves at that moment. Surgery was performed so you could feel better than you did before the surgery. That's the goal to shoot for…and beyond.

35. Hear That Heart

I began reading through the book of Psalms. I was attempting to read five a day for thirty days; sounds easy enough. I'm sure it's because I've been given a new perspective on many subjects since my surgery, but I'm amazed how often the word "heart" is used in the Psalms. It shouldn't be much of a surprise to anyone that I now comprehend these "heart" verses in a whole new light. They now possess a more literal and personal meaning for me. I find myself speaking these verses to my own heart. Hey, if King David could speak to his soul, then I feel complete liberty to do the same to my heart. After all, "A merry heart does good like a medicine…" (Proverbs 17:22), and it "makes a cheerful countenance" (Proverbs15:13) Both of these verses convince me I have nothing to lose and lots to gain by having some bold proclamations toward my own heart and its health. A happy heart, for me, is a healthy heart, and that's cause for a happy person.

So, with that in mind, hear this heart: "The statutes of the Lord are right, rejoicing the *(MY)* heart: the commandment of the Lord is pure, enlightening the *(MY)* eyes" (Psalm 19:8). I don't know anyone who couldn't stand a little lightening up from time to time; that's for sure.

And how about this one: "For our *(MY)* heart shall rejoice in Him, because we *(I)* have trusted in His holy name" (Psalm 33: 21). Trusting in something bigger than me is always good news, not just for my heart, but for my entire well-being. After all, I have witnessed, first hand, how fragile I and my heart really are.

This last one reminds me I cannot change what has passed, but I can boldly face the future: "My flesh and my heart fail; but God is the strength of my heart..." (Psalm 73:26).

36. Having Heart Disease

I was at a follow-up visit with my cardiologist some weeks after my surgery when I first heard the term "heart disease" used in our conversation. Maybe the term was spoken before this, but that was the day it registered in my head as a reference to me. The doctor used it in a third person sort of way saying, "Those with heart disease need to..." I couldn't even hear the rest of what he said. I realized I was one of the "those" he was referring to in his statement. I was immediately offended, because I was being told I had a disease. I got hung up on that "disease" word. My cardiologist had no idea how shocked I was. He just kept on talking. It was just routine conversation to him. Surgery is one thing. It is performed. Patients heal and recuperate. Everyone moves on with life, but, in that word "disease," I did not hear a moving on in it. I heard something that was going to provoke me for the rest of my life. I heard I was going to be battling an enemy in my body from here on out. That one word was a tough pill to swallow. Cardiologists could be more conscious of this, and proceed in their conversations accordingly, maybe seasoning them with a little more grace (Free unsolicited advice, - no charge).

I needed to put a better construction so to speak on this fact that was to accompany me the rest of my life. I couldn't free myself from heart disease, but I could develop both ongoing physical and attitudinal lifestyle changes and habits to give my heart its best fighting chance. Life became a series of decisions, so to speak, that would feed the disease or fight the disease. Some days it's like a game; other days it's more like a battle, both physically and emotionally.

People have always been what make the difference for me. Making a better immediate or long term lifestyle choice always seems clearer and more bearable when the people I love, and I know love me, are considered. I may not be in total control over my physical condition, but I do have a choice of whether I want to be miserable or thankful in it. Each day brings fresh opportunities to make good heart choices or not so good choices, but, I'm here to make them, and they are mine to make.

37. Normal is Wonderful

Many people aspire to be something more than "normal." To most people, being normal may indicate a dull, uneventful existence. It is considered the baseline from which one reaches some kind of higher achievement. Wanting to accomplish something, of course, isn't intrinsically bad; it's just that heart patients, like me, have come to appreciate normalcy as a most welcome friend.

Heart patients view the word normal in a whole different light than non-heart patients. They have been through an event that has knocked their sense of normalcy off course. They are working toward and looking for signs of its return. Encouragement in this endeavor is never overstated.

Many heart patients come out of surgery having to make adjustments in their lifestyles. They may be overweight or have other physical impairments to overcome. Many start exercising in ways they previously never imagined. When they reach a normal weight and blood pressure, it's an occasion for celebration.

Eating habits most likely need some modification. Many patients need to relearn how to eat properly. They have spent years making less than ideal choices, and old habits die hard. When one hears they have reached normal cholesterol levels from making changes in their diet, they truly have accomplished something great.

New medications have probably been recently introduced. This regulation of medications can be both a wearisome and anxious struggle between feeling well and avoiding annoying or debilitating side effects. Feeling normal is not taken lightly.

Through all these adjustments, heart patients like me love and strive to hear the word normal. When I'm told these basic affirmations of being normal, I am encouraged that what I do on a daily basis is giving me the best defense for my hearts future. Normal is wonderful.

38. Good Heart Choices

Once someone has a "heart event," there is no going back. This means from that point forward many daily decisions come down to, "Is this good for my heart?" or "Is this **not** so good for my heart?" Various heart procedures are designed to repair damage that the heart has incurred, but the underlying reasons responsible for that damage, like it or not, should be addressed for the rest of the patient's life.

We like to think of ourselves as well-informed Americans. We all know too much sodium, fat (the "bad" kind of course), and sugar/sweeteners are our hearts' enemies, but to proclaim all these things permanently out of one's diet is unrealistic for most people. My own particular viewpoint is that a heart-healthy lifestyle basically comes down to one decision at a time. Make a better meal choice than you did the meal before. Write up a menu plan with fresh, unprocessed ingredient choices. Most foods are not harmful if kept in moderation. Know what you are planning to eat before you shop so that bad choices won't entice you. Try not to do the bulk of food shopping in the center of the grocery store. The freshest, healthiest choices are predominantly around the periphery of the store. Alter your favorite recipes by substituting lower fat, sodium, and sugar options. Find ways to reduce animal products in your diet. Go ahead; be creative. Read the food labels of some of your favorite packaged foods and try to duplicate and make them yourself without all the additives of the packaged items. Eating healthy does not mean one has to give up on taste. Over the course of time, all these individual choices will add up to a lifestyle change. What I especially like about going one decision at a time is, if one makes a poor decision, another meal is coming soon enough, and a better choice is again available.

39. No Ring (conclusion)

I had not seen my wedding ring since the day of my surgery when I had to take it off. It was now weeks after I had been discharged from the hospital, and my husband had only managed to restore my gold wedding band to my finger. My last hope in finding my diamond ring lay in taking apart our washer and dryer and hopefully discovering it inside one of them. To my frustration, my husband always seemed to have something else more urgent to do than to take apart those machines. We obviously did not share the same emotional attachment to my ring. The day those machines were finally opened up was the day it was settled in my head that my ring was gone, never again to be seen.

Five weeks had now passed since my surgery. It was my birthday. My whole family gathered around our kitchen table to enjoy dinner and dessert. My husband presented me with one small gift wrapped box. The world stopped momentarily. I was convinced there was a new diamond ring sitting in that box. I immediately felt guilty. I had obviously made my husband feel so bad about losing my ring that he felt he had to spend a ton of money on a new one.

Sure enough, inside the box was a new diamond ring and matching wedding band, a definite upgrade from my previous simple solitaire. I was now in tears. The new ring and band were beautiful. I put them on my finger as the dam of emotional flood waters broke. Weeks of pent up anxiety were released. I couldn't hold it back. My family around me all had a good laugh at their mother's expression of "happiness." Hold on; that's not the best part of the story. For the five weeks since my surgery, I had been totally "duped." My husband had decided all the way back on that day I took my ring off in the hospital that it was the perfect opportunity to give it a facelift. He had not lost it. He did an amazing job keeping a secret from a persistent wife. What really impressed me was that it wasn't an entirely new ring. He had taken my original diamond and had it reset into a new setting and band.

My diamond was back on my finger; one more piece of my sense of normalcy had been restored to me. Because it had my original diamond, the new setting was all the more precious to me. His challenge had been to keep me from learning the truth until my birthday-no small feat. All my anxiety was for naught.

After twenty years of marriage, my husband could still surprise me. He endured five weeks of my continual inquiries and pleas without losing his cool or spoiling his secret. Now isn't that one of the cruelest, yet sweetest, stories you ever heard!?

40. Getting in the Steps

One nifty little gadget I've become acquainted with since my surgery is the pedometer. A few years after my recovery, I heard the cardiac center, through which I received my rehabilitation, was giving them away to their patients. They are given as incentive for people to walk and keep track of their daily number of steps taken, distance traveled, and calories burned. I had unsuccessfully tried using some less than impressive pedometers in the past that always seemed to keep inaccurate readings, so I marched back to rehab class to pick up a trustworthy one of my own. Some pedometers, like mine, track your numbers in a seven day memory. Accumulating steps instantly became a new personal game. I compete against myself. A quick search on the internet identifies general activity levels according to the number of daily steps one takes.

One who accumulates less than 5000 steps is generally considered "sedentary." Ouch. That's me on most non-exercise days! 5000 to 7500 steps is considered "somewhat active." 7500 to 10,000 steps is considered "moderately active." Taking over 10,000 steps is considered "active," and this is what an average adult should be shooting for to maintain good cardiac health. Ten thousand steps are equal to walking roughly five miles.

I always considered myself an "active lifestyle" sort of person, so I thought it would be easy to rack up the number of steps corresponding to this lifestyle. I began wearing the pedometer daily. I soon found out that unless I purposely exercised for a minimum of 40 minutes, I didn't achieve the number of steps in a day to qualify as having an active lifestyle. Without daily exercise, I fall into the sedentary category. I was actually amazed at how FEW steps I take as an at-home mom, especially on the days I actually get to remain at home all day. So if I could make a recommendation, get a pedometer and have some fun. Be creative, make goals, and start counting steps for good heart health.

41. Benefits of a Heart Support Group

My first encounter with the Mended Hearts support group is a hazy memory at best. I believe a visitor from the group came to see me in my hospital room my second day out of surgery. I have this foggy recollection of someone trying to tell me they understood how I was feeling and that there was a group of heart patients who met monthly to encourage one another in their recovery and ongoing lifestyle. I managed to thank them for visiting, but what I didn't tell them was that I had no intension of joining any support group.

I am privileged to have a very supportive family and friends who rallied to cover all my extensive needs for me and my family through my entire recovery. I had all the support I needed and/or wanted. My healing process went well.

Fast forward several years later when my youngest child started school. I found myself with some extra time on my hands. I felt drawn back to the cardiac patients in order to encourage them in their own recovery from one who had been in their place. I was confident there were patients out there less fortunate than I had been in receiving encouragement and support in their recovery.

My local hospital welcomed me as a volunteer but directed me to come under the specific training of the Mended Hearts support group there in order to expressly visit heart patients. In order to become better acquainted with the support group under which I was to visit patients, I decided to attend their monthly meetings. I found numerous people with a common thankfulness for life combined with a ready spirit to encourage one another. They each understand, in a most personal way, what the other has experienced. They meet in order to receive regular inspiration for their daily heart healthy choices. They are the real live faces of those who are making those choices. Together, they hold one another accountable, as they gather to arm themselves in the fight against the heart disease they battle in their bodies.

42. Visitors are Visuals

After surgery, patients often wonder what to expect in their immediate and long term recovery. Strength is restored little by little, day by day, step by step. Regaining vitality can be frustrating, and doubts about the future can easily take hold. Visitors who have been former patients themselves can play a huge role in the emotional recovery of a patient. The old adage, "Seeing is believing," is extremely practical for a heart patient. Seeing someone who is physically thriving after their own surgery can deliver a great dose of confidence. Visitors are a visual image of what is possible for the patient.

I love being that positive influence on someone's life. Every time I visit patients at my local hospital, I come away glad I went. I am able to show the patient what is possible for them at a time when they can be feeling the most vulnerable and insecure about their future. Volunteering as a visitor is a commitment to inspire patients to press on to the best recovery and ongoing lifestyle possible. It's very rewarding. We get to do this just by being ourselves; no special talents or skills are needed. Giving of oneself is always a worthwhile investment.

I was personally visited by a Mended Hearts volunteer when I was one day out from surgery. I can't say I was fully coherent or congenial to my visitor. To whoever you were, please accept my apologies. I wasn't quite myself. I put minimal effort into how politely I let the visitor know they could move on to their next patient. In other words, I was a grouchy patient. In my own defense, I think it was too soon after my surgery for an inspirational pep talk.

Now, as I visit patients, I try to be mindful of not over-staying my welcome. I, too, occasionally get treated how I treated my visitor. It's not personal; I understand.

One day, a wife with a husband in surgery was glad to break up the hours in the waiting room to hear a little about my recovery experience. She commented, "My husband should hear your story. He would be encouraged." Of course, I'd be glad to talk with him also.

Another couple in the waiting room recognized me from a previous visit and called me over just for a catch-up kind of a chat and to inquire about cardiac rehabilitation. The husband had not yet gone to the classes and I was able to direct them to those who could help make it happen.

On the recovery floor was a fascinating woman with a cheerful countenance. She had a personal life story I could have listened to for hours. She had a way of welcoming people into her story. I observed how much her family members clearly loved her. I came away thankful for the chance to have met her. I had the impression others left her presence the same way.

I go to the hospital each week to give but always come away having been given to. I start out the visitor and end up the visited.

43. Now I'm Fixed

One misconception I occasionally hear from other recovering heart patients is they believe after heart surgery their heart disease is "fixed." They think they have been given a fresh start to resume a bodily destructive lifestyle - the same one that landed them in surgery to begin with. Some repeat customers to the operating room are ones who went away from their initial operation thinking this way. It is so disappointing to see patients who have to return to the hospital for additional procedures or treatment because of this way of thinking. Truth is, one's valve or arteries may have been repaired, replaced, or bypassed, but the underlying issue causing the breakdown of those vessels may be, and often is, still present. I'm making a distinction here between fixing the actual vessels and fixing the cause of the heart damage. The vessels have been repaired, and good blood flow has been reestablished, but if the patient's lifestyle is not altered or adjusted to one of a heart-healthy one, the vessels will again clog and/or deteriorate.

I realize there will always be those who do take their heart's health seriously and will still find themselves needing additional intervention. I'm not leaving myself out of that category. All of us heart patients, like anyone else, are walking out our life journeys one day at a time with no set guarantees of what the future holds. I just don't desire to receive any additional intervention if it's something I could avoid through proper diet, exercise, and medication. I'm reminding us all: don't take the fact that we "feel" good as a license to cast off restraint and make decisions that will add up to another visit to the emergency room, or worse. We shouldn't cast off restraint because we feel well. That's the wrong thinking. We feel well most likely because we have NOT cast off. Be encouraged to stay diligent in the small daily healthy choices.

44. Consider Yourself Invited

I visited a patient who had just received a stent. He was feeling quite well again and was understandably anxious to go home. With the advancement of technology, more and more people are avoiding major heart surgery by undergoing a less invasive stent procedure. Most stent recipients have about a two day hospital stay compared to surgery patients who stay an average of five to seven days. Many stent recipients receive relief from their chest discomfort almost instantaneously. Not to overwhelm anyone here, but I have visited some patients that have over a dozen stents in them. Stents are placed not only in vessels around the heart but also in other areas where there could be blockage, like the legs. Many stent recipients come and go from the hospital so quickly they frequently miss a visit from a fellow heart patient and are never informed of the availability of a local support group.

As we spoke of the opportunity of attending such a meeting, the patient I was visiting told me he was a regular exerciser at the hospital's cardiac rehabilitation center. I then told him that many of his fellow exercisers there also happened to be members of our support group. He was surprised to learn he already knew some people from the group. I asked him if there was a reason he had never visited the support group meetings. He merely responded he had never thought of it, and no one had ever invited him! "Well." I said, "Consider yourself invited." I was delighted to see him and his wife at our next meeting and ever since. Many people simply don't know a heart support group exists, and how easy it is to attend.

So who are YOU exercising next to that just may not have been invited yet? Go ahead, invite them.

45. Go Ahead Ask Me

Many questions go through a patient's head when they are recovering from surgery. Most of them are for medical professionals to answer. I encourage everyone to ask as many as they can think of to these worthy, experienced experts.

I like to make myself available as the person with the "been there and done that" perspective. I have thought about the uncertainties of the future while lying in bed recuperating. I understand the commitment it takes on a daily basis to get back to good health and the diligence to continue that commitment for the rest of our life. I share the feeling of indebtedness from having to receive so many forms of physical and emotional help from others. I did not like losing my independence and the ability to do basic daily physical functions, even if it was only temporary. I would wonder, as I laid in bed at night, to what extent I would actually physically recover. I understand it's much faster and more convenient to eat fast food rather than buy fresh and cook it oneself from scratch. Even now, I sometimes wake up in the morning thinking I'd rather not exercise today. I, like you, have looked at my own mortality in the face. I've been there too, like you.

Sometimes it's questions about the emotional side of recovery that can be the hardest to ask. Those are the ones that may be difficult to admit or articulate. Maybe we try to ignore thoughts and questions that would make us appear vulnerable or something less than thankful. I say one thing about that, "You're normal." The expression, "There's nothing new under the sun" includes your thoughts. These thoughts are only new to you. You are not alone; others have thought them before you. Every time I am asked to comment on any of these doubts, I get strengthened in my own convictions. Confessing our cares is most of the victory over them. Somewhere in the exposure of them, doubts and fears are broken down and reformed into new strength of character. So, go ahead, ask me about your anxieties. You may not get an expert medical answer, but I will most likely say, "I understand. I've thought about that too, like you."

46. How Long to Normal?

As a heart patient and a frequent visitor of other heart patients, I am often asked, "How long did it take you to feel back to normal again?" I always reply, "That's a loaded question; I don't have a simple answer."

I found my recovery to be a two part process. I don't think it's one a heart patient ever completes. Our recovery becomes a journey through the rest of our lives. There was an initial physical recovery which was obvious to all those around me. I needed lots of rest, but, in between, I regained my strength through rehabilitation classes, walks, and many helpful visits from friends and family. My physical recovery was a steady process, without complications, which brought me through to running my busy household again within weeks after my surgery. A couple months after surgery, I appeared "good as new."

This is about the time my brain kicked in and said, "Okay, now it's my turn." Hence, the second part of my recovery. This emotional recovery is often not so obvious to those around us and can be hard to pin point and describe. It was like all my energy up to that time had gone toward restoring all my physical settings in my body. Suddenly, my brain needed to do some filing, filtering, and processing of its own with all the overload of information it had taken in over my recent history. Just when people around me naturally started backing off and letting me resume my "normal" lifestyle, I found myself still desiring and seeking audible encouragement and companionship. I battled in my brain this feeling of selfishness for wanting continued attention from people who had already given so much time and effort to me. By talking with people, though, I gradually came to an understanding and started practicing in my conversation with others to take the focus off of me and my recovery and project it outward toward others and their edification. (This will be ongoing for the rest of my life, for sure.) Everything is better with talking.

Having people around helped me properly put my physical journey in perspective. It kept me from turning inward on my own "what if this happens or that happens" scenarios and reminded me of how thankful I was to be here. People like my Mom were faithful to tell me often that my heart <u>was</u> in need of repair, and <u>now</u> it was mended. "It's better now than it was," she would say. "Keep up the good work, one decision at a time." Right or wrong, accurate or not, it didn't matter; her words, and others like them, helped and continue to help heal my emotional wounds. They assisted my brain in doing its filing and moving on.

I'm no doctor, but, I would say talking, being around people, and giving of yourself are all key to a heart-healthy recovery, or any recovery for that matter, back to normalcy. It may sound obvious, but too many people find themselves alone in their thoughts, which can have unhealthy results.

I would say my best answer to when back to "normal" is, is when we are back to enjoying the people we have been placed with in this life and giving freely of ourselves to them in some way.
When would you like that to be?

47. Tolerating the Pain

A couple questions I am often asked by those facing their own surgery are, "How painful was your recovery?" and "How did you tolerate the pain after surgery?"

Those questions have as diverse an answer as the number of people answering them. Keep in mind I preface mine with that observation. Patients go into heart surgery under various circumstances; these factors all play a role in the pain experienced after surgery. Simply said, different people tolerate pain differently.

So to answer that question I specifically speak of my own personal recovery and try not to proclaim it as the norm for everyone, but, many find common denominators with my experience.

First of all, as a relief to many, I don't remember experiencing sheer hurtful pain, a kind that would lead one to helpless tears, cries, or anguish. I would describe my experience more like "annoying discomfort." I would want to lie in a certain position, but my incision sites would not allow me that luxury. I would want to move, but I had little strength. I would want to rest, but I couldn't sleep peacefully for any significant length of time. The first couple days after surgery are, as one would imagine, the most uncomfortable. The discomfort eases gradually.

Medications are available to help mask the pain. They play an important role in taking the edge off pain so that one can get the important rest one needs for recovery. If there is one thing I would say it is this: Take your pain medication diligently, in a timely manner, under supervision, especially for the first few days. If you're not able to rest, recovery is impaired. If you don't tolerate a certain medication, ask for and try another. Our bodies need rest as they recover. Amazingly, it's only a matter of days, and one can begin to gradually reduce one's pain medication. I found that the pain medication helped me rest, but it wasn't a peaceful rest. I would have strange, disconnected dreams; I looked forward to easing off the pain medications. I didn't find it necessary to empty my pill container of pain prescription. Take each recovery, of course, one day at a time, realizing once again that everyone is different, but, a couple weeks after surgery I no longer needed or wanted the pain medication.

My chest felt "creaky" for quite some time after surgery. That's my best word to describe it. There was no pain involved. Bones, cartilage, and whatever else inside my incision site seemed to be shifting around a bit as I regained muscular mobility there. I interpreted the creakiness as coming from everything inside my chest finding its proper place and balance once again, and it took a little time. It was another one of those symptoms, like my numb extremities, that gradually faded with time. After ten months to a year, I no longer noticed it.

48. Do Ask and Do Tell

I am not a trained medical professional by any stretch of the imagination and don't claim to be such. My basic premise is to live a heart-healthy, active lifestyle to the best of my ability without additional medicinal aid, and then if I absolutely need that medicinal aid, so be it. Everyone has their own philosophy in this regard; I'm just letting you in on mine for perspective. Let everyone be convinced of where that balance lies between drug intervention and lifestyle modification for their own decisions. I would encourage everyone to make their decisions wisely, having made proper inquiry into them.

I have observed that medicine for heart patients, such as cholesterol fighting drugs, tends to be given at standard dosage amounts based on patient criteria such as age, weight, sex, past history, etc. Some drugs are automatically prescribed on a preventative basis. This works for most people the majority of the time, but not everyone responds to drugs in a standard way. Some people can be extremely sensitive to the form and dosage of certain drugs in their body. Some, like me, would like to know about and try natural alternatives to drugs if possible.

Be encouraged to relay any side-effects or concerns you may have to your doctor until you feel well. Ask questions like, "Could I achieve the same results with a smaller dosage of the drug, or with one that is less expensive?" "What are the long term effects of taking this drug?" "What lifestyle changes can I make to possibly get off or avoid this drug?" You may be pleasantly surprised with the answers you receive, just because you asked.

I have met patients who have gone back to their cardiologist repeatedly because they experienced muscle pain as a side effect of their statin (cholesterol) drug. Sometimes it takes months of trial and error to get to the appropriate drug and dosage that achieves the proper result. This is about your long term health and vitality, so be persistent in getting to a place of feeling and functioning well.

49. The Zipper Club

Heart patients don't walk around with a banner saying, "Talk to me, I'm a heart patient." We blend in with everyone else who is out and about, but occasionally, I strike up a conversation about heart health in the darnedest places. Usually it happens when I am on errands after visiting patients at my local hospital while still wearing my red Mended Hearts volunteer organization visitor polo. My polo has a little red heart logo on it with a zipper line stitched across the center of it. I believe this logo, along with the patient's own scar line left after surgery, is responsible for many heart patients being referred to as members of the "Zipper Club."

I have been stopped by perfect strangers on elevators, in stores, at the bank, at check-out stands, and even on the beach (hard to hide a scar like ours there). They want to share their own heart experience, tell me about a friend of theirs, ask where they could obtain additional information, or just ask what the logo represents.

Those of us who have recovered from major heart surgery have a lot of hope and encouragement to offer people. We have been physically brought down to square one after surgery and have rebuilt a working relationship again with our bodies. It can be a long process; it can take months of rehabilitation to return to a sense of normalcy in one's life, and, it doesn't stop there. Diligence and encouragement must persist if we are to maintain a healthy lifestyle. I consider it a privilege when I get an opportunity to exchange encouragement with others. It's not the best of circumstances that lead many to become members of the "Zipper Club." Actually, all who desire to achieve and/or maintain a heart healthy lifestyle are welcome at any Mended Hearts meeting, whether they have had surgery or not. The logo is a light-hearted expression of a serious situation, and sometimes that's a good place to initiate an opportunity to encourage and strengthen others making daily choices on the course of promoting one's heart health.

50. People, Give, Outside

I am involved in a program through Mended Hearts, Inc., which acts as a type of command center for heart patients to electronically connect with one another. Patients or caretakers contact the Mended Hearts website with a brief synopsis of their situation and request information about the organization or encouragement from other heart patients. Requests to connect with other heart patients are then sent out to a network of trained volunteers from all over the country through the email who may choose to answer the inquiry. For example, I am a mother who was in my 40's when I underwent bypass surgery. I respond to requests made by other women in similar circumstances.

I find myself repeating three very basic yet significant pieces of advice which don't require an investment of money or any special skills. First of all, <u>get around people</u>... friends, family, children, a support, hobby, or church group. The idea is to avoid spending the majority of your time alone. Having people around, helps keep you from getting introspective on yourself. You are forced to think outward about others. None of your friends and family will be opposed to you thinking about them; they may be pleasantly surprised by the attention going in their direction.

This leads right into my second piece of advice: <u>Find opportunities to give</u>. Even though you need extra physical attention during this time, get the focus off yourself as often as you can. It doesn't have to be a grand, thought-out plan. It may be as simple as calling a friend to inquire about them or inviting a child to sit beside you in order to read them a story. Invite a friend to join you for rehabilitation class and treat them to a healthy smoothie afterwards. The simpler the idea, the more likely it will happen.

Lastly, get outside. It sounds insignificant, but there's something to be said about getting fresh air. I think fresh outdoor air is extremely under-rated. It has a way of clearing the thoughts and ushering in fresh perspectives. Pressing issues become less stressful and easier to face after a nice walk in the neighborhood. Walking at the indoor mall just doesn't produce the same results, but if it's your only option sometimes, don't pass it up.

One of my favorite ways of taking all three pieces of my own advice at once is to (1) grab a friend, (2) give them my attention, and (3) take a walk outside together (3). It will do both of you good. Hopefully, you'll start a good, long-term habit and relationship.

Take it From Here

If you have gotten to this page, I presume I have accompanied you through a good chunk of your own personal recovery, or at least given you some insight into what you may experience. Either way, my intent for writing this book has been realized. I hope this small book has given some lasting encouragement to heart patients in each of their unique circumstances.

One main point I hope I made is that each heart procedure recovery is ongoing. It continues out into the rest of our lives. That's just the way it is. Whether we like it or not doesn't negate the fact. It's good to have some people/friends around that understand this. They will help, mostly through verbal encouragement, to keep you tracking along.

The last entry has set you up with my parting piece of advice to be taken away and practiced. Go forth and apply it to your surroundings and situations as you continue your own heart health journey. I believe the creative possibilities are limitless. I love congratulating others in their own little victories. My wish is that we could all continue learning to care for our primary stewardship - that of caring for our own body - in order to maintain good heart health, give freely to others, and avoid future hospital stays.

My very best wishes to you all.

About the Author

Diane Caputo faced open heart surgery after suddenly suffering two heart attacks and undergoing a less than successful stent procedure. In a matter of a few short days, she went from a perfectly healthy, active mother, running a busy household of eight young children, to someone requiring assistance for the smallest of needs. After surgery she had to start from ground zero, physically, and work her way back to what she considered her "normal" lifestyle.

Diane has found that many cardiac patients share similarities with her own experiences in both their physical and emotional recoveries. She felt the need to get the message out to other patients that they are not alone, nor is what they experience unusual or abnormal.

Since her surgery, Diane has regained her active lifestyle and continually seeks practical ways of nurturing a heart-healthy lifestyle for herself and her family. She enjoys creating and modifying recipes using wholesome ingredients. She likes all types of exercise including jogging, Pilates, aerobics, gardening, hiking, or just walking with a friend.

Diane is an accredited visitor for Mended Hearts, Inc., at her local hospital in Olympia, WA. Mended Hearts is a nationwide network of support groups made up of people who have experienced some form of heart event. For more information, visit their website at: MendedHearts.org.

Made in the USA
San Bernardino, CA
10 July 2015